Teen Girl's Survival Guide

Navigating Adolescence: A Teen Girl's Handbook for Thriving in a Complex World

Sarah Mackenzie

Copyright ©

Sarah Mackenzie

© 2024 United Kingdom

Gratitude

Dear Amazing Teen Girl,

I want to take a moment to express my deepest gratitude to you for choosing to embark on this journey with me through the pages of the "Teen Girl's Survival Guide."

Your decision to bring this book into your life means the world to me.

By investing in yourself and your growth, you're demonstrating incredible strength and courage.

You're choosing to navigate the twists and turns of adolescence with wisdom and resilience, and that's truly inspiring.

As you dive into the chapters of this guide, my hope is that you'll find nuggets of wisdom, encouragement, and practical advice that resonate with you deeply.

May these words serve as a compass, guiding you through the challenges and celebrating the victories that lie ahead.

Thank you for trusting me to be a part of your journey.

Remember, you are capable, you are worthy, and you are never alone.

Table of Contents

Introduction

Hey there, beautiful soul!

Welcome to the Teen Girl's Survival Guide—a sanctuary of wisdom, wit, and warmth crafted just for you.

Whether you're flipping through these pages with excitement, curiosity, or maybe even a hint of trepidation, know that you've found a safe space here—a place where you can laugh, learn, and grow.

Teenagehood—it's a wild ride, isn't it? From the dizzying highs of newfound freedoms to the heart-wrenching lows of uncertainty and self-doubt, navigating this transformative journey can sometimes feel like riding a rollercoaster blindfolded. But fear not, my friend, for you are not alone.

In these pages, I've poured my heart and soul into creating a roadmap—a guiding light to help you navigate the twists and turns of adolescence with grace, grit, and a whole lot of girl power.

Whether you're grappling with the mysteries of puberty, wrestling with the complexities of friendship, or charting the uncharted waters of love and self-discovery, consider this book your trusty companion—the ultimate toolkit for thriving in the teen years.

So, why a survival guide for teen girls, you might ask? Well, because let's face it—being a teenage girl in today's world comes with its fair share of challenges. From the pressures of social media perfection to the relentless pursuit of academic excellence, the expectations placed upon teen girls like you can sometimes feel suffocating.

But here's the thing: you are so much more than the sum of your grades, your likes, or your followers. You are a force to be reckoned with—a fiercely fabulous individual with infinite potential.

Throughout these pages, we'll embark on a journey of self-discovery—a quest to uncover the unique magic that lies within you.

We'll dive deep into the murky waters of puberty, unpacking the mysteries of your changing body with honesty and humor.

We'll explore the intricacies of friendship—the joys, the tears, and everything in between—learning how to build authentic connections that nourish your soul.

We'll tackle the tough stuff too—addressing anxiety, self-esteem struggles, and the myriad challenges that life throws our way.

But most importantly, we'll celebrate YOU—your quirks, your dreams, your beautiful imperfections.

Because here's the secret, my dear: you are already enough, just as you are. You don't need to be perfect, you just need to be you.

So, whether you're curled up in your favorite spot with a cup of tea, or sneakily reading under the covers with a flashlight (hey, no judgment here!), know that you're embarking on an incredible adventure—one filled with laughter, learning, and limitless possibilities.

So buckle up, darling, and get ready to embark on the ride of a lifetime. Because with this survival guide by your side, there's nothing you can't handle.

You've got this.

Understanding Your Unique Identity

You're not just another face in the crowd or a name on a class roster—you're a masterpiece in the making, a tapestry woven with threads of passion, quirks, and dreams.

Your favorite hobbies, your quirky habits, your wildest aspirations—they all come together to create the vibrant mosaic of your personality.

But here's the thing: discovering your unique identity isn't always a piece of cake. In a world where conformity often feels like the norm, it's easy to lose sight of what makes you truly special.

That's why it's essential to take the time to explore every nook and cranny of your soul—to embrace the quirks, celebrate the passions, and honor the dreams that set your heart on fire.

So, where do you start on this exhilarating journey of self-discovery? Begin by tuning in to your inner voice—the whisper of your heart that knows you better than anyone else.

What are you passionate about? What makes your heart sing and your spirit soar?

Whether it's writing poetry, belting out tunes in the shower, or exploring the great outdoors, your passions are the breadcrumbs that lead you back to your true self.

Next, take a moment to reflect on your values—the guiding principles that shape your decisions and define who you are as a person.

What matters most to you? Is it kindness, integrity, creativity, or something else entirely?

Your values are the compass that points you in the direction of your true north, helping you navigate life's twists and turns with grace and authenticity.

And finally, don't be afraid to embrace the quirks that make you uniquely you. Maybe you're a bookworm who can recite Harry Potter quotes by heart, or perhaps you're a budding scientist with a

penchant for conducting experiments in your backyard.

Whatever makes you different, wear it like a badge of honor—because it's those quirks that make you shine brightest in a world full of ordinary.

So, my dear, embrace your uniqueness with open arms. Celebrate the quirks, honor the passions, and trust that the journey of self-discovery is one of the most beautiful adventures life has to offer.

You're a masterpiece in the making, and the world is waiting with bated breath to see the masterpiece you become.

Setting Goals and Dreams

Setting goals and dreaming big isn't just about wishful thinking—it's about laying the groundwork for a future that sets your soul on fire.

Whether you dream of becoming a world-renowned artist, a groundbreaking scientist, or a champion of social justice, your goals are the stepping stones that pave the path to your wildest dreams.

So, where do you begin on this exhilarating journey of goal-setting and dream-chasing? Let's break it down into bite-sized steps:

Dream Big

Close your eyes and imagine the world of your dreams. What does it look like?

What does it feel like? Whether it's traveling the globe, starting your own business, or making a difference in your community, let your imagination run wild.

Remember, there are no limits to what you can achieve—except the limits you place on yourself.

Get Specific

Once you've conjured up your dream destination, it's time to map out the route to get there.

Break down your big dreams into smaller, actionable goals—think of them as mini-adventures along the way. Want to become a published author? Start by setting a goal to write a certain number of pages or chapters each week.

Dreaming of running a marathon? Set a goal to increase your mileage by a certain distance each month. The key is to make your goals specific, measurable, and achievable.

Stay Flexible

Life is like a rollercoaster—full of unexpected twists and turns. While it's important to set goals and chart your course, it's equally important to stay flexible and adapt to the inevitable changes along the way.

If a roadblock pops up or a detour presents itself, don't get discouraged—view it as an opportunity to recalibrate your route and discover new paths to success.

Stay Inspired

Chasing your dreams can sometimes feel like a marathon, not a sprint. That's why it's essential to stay inspired along the way.

Surround yourself with people who believe in you, immerse yourself in activities that fuel your passion, and never underestimate the power of a good pep talk (even if it's just from yourself!).

And remember, it's okay to take breaks, recharge your batteries, and indulge in a little self-care along the way.

Celebrate Your Victories

Every step forward, no matter how small, is a victory worth celebrating.

Whether you reach a major milestone or simply make progress toward your goals, take a moment to pat yourself on the back and revel in your accomplishments.

You're a rockstar, and you deserve to bask in the glow of your own awesomeness.

So, my dear dreamer, let your goals be your guiding stars and your dreams be your North Star.

With passion, perseverance, and a sprinkle of pixie dust, there's no limit to how far you can go and how high you can soar.

Dream big, aim high, and remember—you've got this!

Navigating the Ups and Downs of Puberty

Your Changing Body: What to Expect

Puberty—it's a rollercoaster of changes, both inside and out. From mood swings to growth spurts, acne breakouts to newfound curves, navigating this transformative journey can sometimes feel like riding a wave in a stormy sea.

But fear not, my friend, for you are not alone. In fact, you're in excellent company—millions of girls around the world are experiencing the very same changes as you read these words.

So, how do you navigate the ups and downs of puberty with grace, grit, and a whole lot of girl power? Well, let's get right into it.

Educate Yourself

Knowledge is power, especially when it comes to understanding what's happening to your body during puberty.

Take the time to educate yourself about the changes you can expect to experience—from menstruation to breast development to hormonal fluctuations.

There are plenty of reliable resources available, from trusted websites to books written specifically for teens like you.

Embrace the Changes

Repeat after me: change is beautiful. Sure, puberty might come with its fair share of awkward moments and uncomfortable conversations, but it's also a sign that your body is doing exactly what it's supposed to do—growing, evolving, and blossoming into the incredible woman you're destined to become.

So embrace the changes, celebrate your body, and remember that beauty comes in all shapes, sizes, and stages of development.

Practice Self-Care

Puberty can be a rollercoaster of emotions, from exhilarating highs to heart-wrenching lows. That's why it's essential to prioritize self-care and nurture your mental and emotional well-being. Whether it's journaling, practicing mindfulness, or indulging in your favorite hobbies, find activities that help you feel grounded, centered, and at peace with yourself.

Seek Support

Remember, you don't have to navigate the ups and downs of puberty alone. Reach out to trusted adults—whether it's a parent, guardian, teacher, or school counselor—and lean on them for support, guidance, and reassurance.

And don't forget about your friends—they're experiencing many of the same changes as you, and together, you can laugh, cry, and commiserate your way through puberty's wild ride.

Celebrate Your Uniqueness

Last but not least, celebrate what makes you uniquely you. Whether it's your quirky sense of humor, your infectious laughter, or your killer dance moves, embrace the qualities that make you shine like the superstar you are.

Always bear in mind that there's no one else in the world quite like you, and that's something worth celebrating every single day.

The following are some of the changes to expect in your body when puberty sets in:

Breast Development: One of the most noticeable changes during puberty is breast development.

You may notice that your breasts start to grow, sometimes starting as small bumps beneath your nipples.

As you continue to mature, your breasts will gradually take on different shapes and sizes, and you might experience tenderness or sensitivity.

Menstruation: Ah, the infamous period—perhaps the most talked-about aspect of puberty. Menstruation, or your monthly period, marks the beginning of your reproductive years.

You'll experience a monthly cycle where your uterus sheds its lining, resulting in bleeding that typically lasts for a few days.

Along with menstruation, you may also experience symptoms like cramping, bloating, and mood swings.

Body Hair: Get ready to welcome some new guests to the party—body hair! During puberty, you'll start to notice hair sprouting in new places, such as your underarms, legs, and pubic area.

This is completely normal and happens as a result of hormonal changes in your body. You can choose to groom or remove this hair if you wish, but remember, it's entirely up to you and what makes you feel comfortable and confident.

Acne: Ah, acne—the bane of many teenagers' existence. As your hormones kick into high gear during puberty, you may notice an increase in oil production on your skin, leading to breakouts and pimples.

While acne can be frustrating, it's essential to remember that it's a natural part of puberty and doesn't define your worth or beauty.

 With proper skincare and self-care practices, you can keep those pesky pimples at bay and embrace your glowing, radiant skin.

Growth Spurts: Get ready to reach new heights—literally! During puberty, you'll experience rapid growth spurts as your bones and muscles grow and develop. You may find yourself shooting up several inches in a short period, which can sometimes lead to feelings of clumsiness or awkwardness.

Embrace these changes with open arms and remember that growing pains are just a sign that your body is doing exactly what it's supposed to do—grow and thrive.

Emotional Changes: Along with physical changes, puberty also brings a whirlwind of emotional changes. You may find yourself experiencing mood swings, intense emotions, and newfound interests or passions.

This is all part of the journey of self-discovery and learning to navigate your ever-changing emotions with grace and resilience.

So, my dear, incredible girl, embrace these changes with open arms and a fierce spirit.

Puberty may bring its fair share of ups and downs, but it's also a beautiful journey of self-discovery, growth, and empowerment. Remember, you are strong, you are beautiful, and you are perfectly imperfect just the way you are.

Self-Care and Hygiene Practices for Teen Girls During Puberty

Self-Care Practices

Nourish Your Body: Your body is a temple, and it deserves to be treated with love and respect.

During puberty, your body is undergoing rapid changes, so it's essential to fuel it with nutritious foods that support your growth and development.

Load up on fruits, veggies, whole grains, and lean proteins, and remember to stay hydrated by drinking plenty of water throughout the day.

Move Your Body: Exercise isn't just about burning calories—it's about celebrating the incredible capabilities of your body and nourishing your soul.

Find activities that bring you joy and make you feel alive, whether it's dancing, swimming, yoga, or simply taking a leisurely stroll through nature.

Moving your body releases endorphins, boosts your mood, and helps you feel strong and empowered from the inside out.

Prioritize Sleep: Oh, the sweet embrace of slumber—there's nothing quite like it! Getting enough sleep is crucial for your physical, emotional, and mental well-being, especially during puberty when your body is working overtime to support your growth and development.

Aim for 8-10 hours of quality sleep each night, and create a relaxing bedtime routine to help you unwind and prepare for a restful night's sleep.

Practice Mindfulness: In a world filled with distractions and noise, finding moments of peace and stillness is more important than ever.

Mindfulness practices like meditation, deep breathing, and journaling can help you quiet the chatter of your mind, tune into your inner wisdom, and cultivate a sense of calm and clarity amidst the chaos of puberty.

Unplug and Recharge: While technology can be a powerful tool for connection and learning, it's essential to unplug and disconnect from screens regularly to give your mind and body a much-needed break.

Set boundaries around screen time, especially before bedtime, and prioritize activities that nourish your soul and feed your creativity, whether it's reading a book, spending time in nature, or getting crafty with DIY projects.

Connect with Others: Puberty can sometimes feel like a lonely journey, but you're not alone. Reach out to trusted friends, family members, or mentors who can offer support, guidance, and a listening ear when you need it most. Surround yourself with people who lift you up, cheer you on, and remind you of your incredible worth and potential.

Celebrate Your Wins: Every step forward, no matter how small, is a victory worth celebrating.

Whether you ace a test, conquer a fear, or simply make it through a challenging day, take a moment to pat yourself on the back and acknowledge your accomplishments.

Personal Hygiene Practices

Puberty is a time of incredible growth and change, and taking care of your body is an essential part of feeling confident and comfortable in your own skin.

So, let's explore some self-hygiene practices tailored just for you:

Daily Showering: Daily showers are essential for keeping your body clean and fresh, especially during puberty when your hormones are in full swing.

Make it a habit to shower at least once a day, using a mild soap or body wash to cleanse your skin. Pay special attention to areas that tend to sweat more, like your underarms and groin, and be sure to rinse thoroughly to remove any traces of soap or shampoo.

Hair Care: Whether you have long, flowing locks or a cute pixie cut, taking care of your hair is an important part of your self-hygiene routine.

Wash your hair regularly with a gentle shampoo and conditioner that's suited to your hair type, and be sure to rinse thoroughly to remove any product buildup. If you use styling tools or products, be mindful of how often you use them and give your hair regular breaks to air dry and rest.

Oral Hygiene: A bright, confident smile is one of your best accessories, so be sure to take care of those pearly whites!

Brush your teeth at least twice a day, using a fluoride toothpaste and a soft-bristled toothbrush.

Don't forget to floss daily to remove plaque and food particles from between your teeth, and consider using a mouthwash for added freshness and protection against cavities.

Menstrual Hygiene: Ah, periods—the not-so-glamorous side of puberty. But fear not, my friend, because managing your menstrual hygiene is easier than ever with a few simple tips and tricks.

Stock up on menstrual products like pads, tampons, or menstrual cups, and choose the option that feels most comfortable and convenient for you.

Change your menstrual products regularly to prevent leaks and odors, and be sure to wash your hands before and after handling them.

Underarm Care: As your body undergoes hormonal changes during puberty, you may notice an increase in sweat and body odor, especially in your underarms.

Combat this by washing your underarms daily with soap and water, and consider using a deodorant or antiperspirant to keep odor and sweat at bay.

Look for products that are gentle on your skin and free from harsh chemicals, and reapply as needed throughout the day.

Intimate Hygiene: Last but not least, taking care of your intimate areas is crucial for maintaining overall hygiene and comfort.

Wash your vulva and surrounding areas with warm water and a mild, fragrance-free soap, and be sure to rinse thoroughly to remove any traces of soap or cleanser.

Avoid douching or using harsh, scented products in your intimate area, as these can disrupt the natural balance of bacteria and lead to irritation or infections.

self-hygiene is all about feeling confident, comfortable, and empowered in your own skin.

Embrace these self-care practices with open arms, and know that taking care of your body is an act of self-love and self-respect.

Building Confidence and Self-Esteem

Practice Self-Compassion

The journey to confidence and self-esteem begins with self-compassion—the art of treating yourself with kindness, understanding, and acceptance, especially during challenging times.

Be gentle with yourself, my friend, and remember that it's okay to make mistakes, stumble, and fall along the way. Treat yourself as you would treat your best friend—with love, compassion, and unwavering support.

Challenge Negative Thoughts

Your mind is a powerful tool, and sometimes it can be your own worst enemy, filling your head with doubts, insecurities, and negative self-talk.

But here's the thing: you have the power to challenge those negative thoughts and rewrite the script.

The next time you catch yourself thinking something negative about yourself, pause, and ask yourself, "Is this thought true? Is it helpful? Is it kind?" If the answer is no, replace it with a positive affirmation or mantra that uplifts and empowers you.

Below are some positive affirmations and mantras that you can apply:

"I am enough, just as I am."

"I believe in myself and my abilities."

"I am worthy of love, respect, and success."

"I embrace my imperfections and celebrate my uniqueness."

"I trust in my inner wisdom to guide me through challenges."

"I am strong, resilient, and capable of overcoming any obstacle."

"I am worthy of all the good things life has to offer."

"I am confident in my choices and decisions."

"I am beautiful, inside and out."

"I am the architect of my own destiny, and I choose to create a life filled with joy, love, and abundance."

Feel free to choose the affirmations that resonate most with you, or create your own personalized mantras that speak directly to your heart and soul.

The power of positive affirmations lies in their ability to shift your mindset and beliefs, so repeat them often and with conviction to amplify their impact on your confidence and self-esteem.

Set Realistic Goals

Goal-setting isn't just about achieving external success—it's about building confidence and self-esteem from the inside out.

Set realistic, achievable goals that align with your values, passions, and strengths, and celebrate your progress along the way. Whether it's acing a test, learning a new skill, or stepping out of your comfort zone, each step forward is a victory worth celebrating and a testament to your incredible resilience and determination.

Celebrate Your Strengths

You, my dear, are a powerhouse of talent, creativity, and potential, and it's time to celebrate the incredible strengths that make you uniquely you.

Take a moment to reflect on your talents, passions, and accomplishments, and celebrate the qualities that make you shine like the superstar you are. Whether you're a gifted artist, a natural leader, or a compassionate friend, each of your strengths is a gift to be cherished and celebrated.

Surround Yourself with Positive Influences:

They say that you become the average of the five people you spend the most time with, so choose your tribe wisely, my friend.

Surround yourself with people who lift you up, inspire you, and believe in your dreams—people who see your potential even when you can't see it yourself. Seek out mentors, role models, and friends who embody the confidence and self-esteem you aspire to

cultivate, and let their light guide you on your journey.

Practice Self-Care

Taking care of yourself isn't just a luxury—it's a necessity, especially during puberty when your body and mind are undergoing rapid changes.

Make self-care a priority in your daily routine, whether it's practicing mindfulness, indulging in your favorite hobbies, or spending time in nature. Nurture your body, mind, and soul with activities that replenish your energy, boost your mood, and remind you of your inherent worth and value.

Celebrate Your Uniqueness

Last but not least, embrace what makes you uniquely you. You are a masterpiece in the making, a dazzling kaleidoscope of quirks, passions, and dreams, and there is no one else in the world quite like you.

Celebrate your quirks, honor your passions, and trust that the world needs your unique light and magic now more than ever.

Making Genuine Friends and Connections

While making friends is undoubtedly one of life's greatest joys, it's also important to choose your connections wisely and surround yourself with people who uplift and inspire you.

So, let's explore some strategies to help you avoid making the wrong friends who may influence you negatively:

Know Your Values:

The first step in choosing the right friends is knowing what matters most to you. Take some time to reflect on your values, beliefs, and priorities in life.

What kind of person do you aspire to be? What qualities do you admire in others?

By clarifying your values, you'll have a clear compass to guide you in choosing friends who align with your principles and support your journey.

Trust Your Instincts:

Your gut instinct is a powerful tool, so don't ignore it! If something feels off about a potential friend or if you find yourself feeling uncomfortable in their presence, trust your instincts and proceed with caution.

Pay attention to how you feel when you're around them—do they uplift and energize you, or do they drain your energy and make you feel uneasy?

Look for Red Flags:

While everyone has flaws and imperfections, there are certain behaviors that should raise a red flag when it comes to potential friends.

Watch out for signs of manipulation, dishonesty, or disrespect, and steer clear of individuals who exhibit these behaviors. Remember, true friendship is built on a foundation of trust, respect, and mutual support.

Observe Their Character:

Actions speak louder than words, so pay attention to how potential friends treat others and navigate the world around them. Are they kind, compassionate, and considerate of others' feelings?

Do they demonstrate integrity, honesty, and authenticity in their words and actions? Surround yourself with people who embody the qualities you admire and aspire to cultivate in yourself.

Set Boundaries:

Healthy friendships are built on a foundation of mutual respect and understanding, which means setting boundaries is essential. Be clear about your values, priorities, and limits, and communicate them openly and honestly with your friends.

If someone consistently crosses your boundaries or disrespects your values, don't be afraid to assert yourself and reevaluate the relationship.

Seek Out Positive Influences:

Surround yourself with people who inspire you, uplift you, and bring out the best in you.

Seek out friends who share your interests, passions, and goals, and who encourage you to pursue your dreams with passion and determination. Positive influences can have a profound impact on your life, so choose your friends wisely and invest in relationships that nourish your soul and ignite your spirit.

Be Your Own Best Friend:

Last but not least, remember that the most important relationship you'll ever have is the one you have with yourself.

Be your own best friend, treat yourself with kindness and compassion, and honor your worth and value as a unique and incredible individual. When you cultivate a strong sense of self-love and self-respect, you'll naturally attract friends who mirror those qualities and support you on your journey.

Be Authentic:

The key to making genuine connections lies in authenticity—being true to yourself and allowing others to see the real you.

Instead of trying to fit into a mold or be someone you're not, embrace your quirks, passions, and unique qualities. When you show up as your authentic self, you attract like-minded individuals who appreciate you for who you truly are.

Show Empathy:

Empathy is the secret sauce that fuels genuine connections—it's the ability to understand and share the feelings of others, to walk in their shoes and see the world through their eyes.

Practice empathy by listening actively, showing compassion, and putting yourself in the shoes of others. When you approach friendships with empathy and kindness, you create a safe and nurturing space for genuine connections to flourish.

Find Common Ground:

Shared interests and experiences are the building blocks of friendship, so seek out opportunities to connect with others who share your passions and hobbies.

Whether it's joining a sports team, a club, or a volunteer organization, finding common ground can help you bond with others and lay the foundation for meaningful connections.

Be a Good Listener:

In a world filled with noise and distractions, being a good listener is a rare and precious gift.

Practice the art of active listening by giving your full attention to the person you're talking to, asking open-ended questions, and showing genuine interest in what they have to say.

When you listen with an open heart and an open mind, you create space for deeper, more authentic conversations to unfold.

Be Vulnerable:

Vulnerability is the secret ingredient that deepens connections and fosters intimacy—it's the willingness to show your true colors, flaws and all, and let others see the raw, unfiltered version of yourself.

 Share your hopes, fears, dreams, and insecurities with trusted friends, and allow yourself to be seen and accepted for who you truly are.

When you embrace vulnerability, you invite others to do the same, creating bonds that are built on trust, authenticity, and mutual respect.

Be Supportive:

True friendship is a two-way street, built on a foundation of trust, respect, and support.

Be there for your friends during both the good times and the bad, offering a listening ear, a shoulder to lean on, and a hand to hold whenever they need it.

Celebrate their successes, lift them up during challenges, and let them know that you've always got their back, no matter what.

Be Open to New Connections:

Genuine friendships can blossom in the most unexpected places, so keep an open mind and an open heart as you navigate the social landscape of puberty.

Strike up conversations with new people, attend social events and gatherings, and be open to making connections with individuals from all walks of life.

You never know—you might just meet your next best friend in the most unlikely of places.

Choosing the right friends is a journey of self-discovery, growth, and empowerment, and with a little wisdom and discernment, you can create a vibrant connections and friendships that enrich your life in countless ways.

Dealing with Drama and Conflict

While drama and conflict are a natural part of life, learning how to navigate them with poise and confidence can help you emerge stronger, wiser, and more empowered than ever.

So, let's explore some strategies to help you deal with drama and conflict like a boss:

Stay Calm:

When drama rears its head or conflict arises, it's easy to let your emotions run wild and react impulsively. But here's the secret: staying calm is your superpower. Take a deep breath, count to ten, and give yourself a moment to collect your thoughts and emotions before responding.

Remember, you are the master of your reactions, and responding from a place of calm and clarity will help you navigate the situation with grace and confidence.

Communicate Effectively:

Clear, open communication is the key to resolving conflicts and diffusing drama. Express yourself honestly and assertively, using "I" statements to share your thoughts, feelings, and needs without blaming or accusing others.

Listen actively to the perspectives of others, and strive to understand their point of view with empathy and compassion.

By fostering open, honest communication, you can build bridges of understanding and find common ground even in the midst of conflict.

Here are some examples of how you can use "I" statements in various situations:

Expressing Feelings:

Instead of: "You always make me feel ignored."

Use "I" statement: "I feel ignored when I'm not included in the conversation."

Addressing Behavior:

Instead of: "You never listen to me."

Use "I" statement: "I feel unheard when I don't feel like my thoughts are being acknowledged."

Stating Needs:

Instead of: "You never help with chores."

Use "I" statement: "I need help with chores, and it would mean a lot to me if we could divide them evenly."

Expressing Disagreement:

Instead of: "You're wrong about this."

Use "I" statement: "I see things differently, and I have a different perspective on this issue."

Setting Boundaries:

Instead of: "You always invade my personal space."

Use "I" statement: "I need my personal space respected, and it makes me uncomfortable when boundaries are crossed."

Expressing Appreciation:

Instead of: "You're always so helpful."

Use "I" statement: "I appreciate your help, and it means a lot to me when you support me in this way."

Remember, the key to effective communication with "I" statements is to focus on your own thoughts, feelings, and needs without placing blame or accusing others.

By using "I" statements, you can express yourself assertively while fostering understanding and empathy in your interactions with others.

Choose Your Battles:

Not every drama is worth engaging in, and not every conflict is worth fighting. Before getting drawn into drama or conflict, ask yourself, "Is this worth my time and energy?"

Consider whether the situation is something you can influence or control, and whether engaging will ultimately serve your best interests.

Sometimes, the best course of action is to let go of the drama and focus on what truly matters to you.

Set Boundaries:

Healthy boundaries are essential for protecting your well-being and preserving your peace of mind.

Be clear about your limits, values, and priorities, and assert yourself confidently when those boundaries are crossed. Whether it's saying no to drama-filled situations or removing yourself from toxic relationships, prioritize your own mental and emotional health above all else.

Seek Support:

Dealing with drama and conflict can sometimes feel overwhelming, so don't hesitate to reach out for support when you need it.

Lean on trusted friends, family members, or mentors who can offer perspective, guidance, and a listening ear. Sometimes, simply talking through your feelings with a supportive confidant can help you gain clarity and find solutions to navigate the situation effectively.

Learn and Grow:

Every experience, whether positive or negative, is an opportunity for growth and learning.

Instead of dwelling on past conflicts or getting caught up in drama, focus on what you can learn from the situation and how you can grow stronger as a result.

Use each experience as a stepping stone to becoming the confident, resilient, and empowered individual you were meant to be.

Drama and conflict may be a part of life, but with the right mindset and tools, you can navigate them with grace, resilience, and unshakeable confidence.

Managing Fights with Friends

Understanding the Dynamics:

Recognize Normalcy: First things first, it's essential to recognize that conflicts with friends are a normal part of any relationship.

Disagreements, misunderstandings, and hurt feelings happen from time to time, and they don't necessarily mean the end of a friendship.

Understanding this can help ease some of the stress and anxiety that often accompanies conflicts.

Communication Breakdown: Many friend conflicts stem from miscommunication or a lack of understanding.

Sometimes, what one person says or does may be interpreted differently by another, leading to hurt feelings or resentment.

Recognizing the role that communication plays in conflicts can help you approach them with a clearer understanding of what went wrong.

Handling Conflicts:

Take a Step Back: When conflicts arise, it can be tempting to react impulsively or emotionally.

However, taking a step back to cool off and gather your thoughts can be incredibly beneficial.

Give yourself some time and space to process your feelings before attempting to address the conflict with your friend.

Express Your Feelings: When you're ready, approach your friend in a calm and respectful manner to express how you're feeling. Use "I" statements to share your thoughts and emotions without placing blame or accusing them.

For example, instead of saying, "You always ignore me," try saying, "I feel hurt when I don't hear from you."

Listen with Empathy: Remember that conflicts involve two people, each with their own perspective and feelings.

Practice active listening by giving your friend the opportunity to share their side of the story without interrupting or getting defensive. Try to empathize with their feelings and understand where they're coming from, even if you don't agree with them.

Find Common Ground: Look for areas of agreement or common ground that you can build upon to resolve the conflict.

Focus on finding solutions rather than assigning blame, and work together with your friend to come up with mutually beneficial resolutions that address both of your needs and concerns.

Apologize and Forgive: If you've played a role in the conflict, take responsibility for your actions and apologize sincerely to your friend. Likewise, be open to forgiving your friend if they apologize to you.

Note that forgiveness doesn't mean forgetting or condoning hurtful behavior—it means letting go of resentment and moving forward with a renewed sense of trust and understanding.

Moving Forward:

Learn and Grow: Every conflict presents an opportunity for growth and learning. Reflect on what you've learned from the experience, and use it to inform how you approach future conflicts and navigate your friendships with greater empathy, resilience, and maturity.

Let Go of Resentment: Holding onto resentment or grudges will only weigh you down and prevent you from moving forward. Practice forgiveness and let go of any lingering resentment towards your friend, even if the conflict wasn't fully resolved.

Forgiveness is a gift you give yourself, and it's essential for your own emotional well-being and peace of mind.

Focus on the Positive: Instead of dwelling on the conflict, focus on the positive aspects of your friendship and the things you value and appreciate about your friend.

Celebrate the strengths and qualities that make your friendship special, and nurture those bonds with kindness, understanding, and mutual respect.

Embracing Growth:

Embrace Growth: Conflict is a natural part of any relationship, and it offers valuable opportunities for personal and interpersonal growth. Embrace the challenges and opportunities that come with navigating conflicts in your friendships, and use them as catalysts for self-discovery, empathy, and resilience.

Seek Resolution: While conflicts may be inevitable, they don't have to define your friendships.

Seek resolution and reconciliation with your friends whenever possible, and prioritize building stronger, healthier relationships based on trust, respect, and understanding.

Remember Your Worth: Above all, remember that you are worthy of friendships that uplift, support, and nourish your soul. Don't settle for relationships that bring you down or make you feel less than your best self.

Surround yourself with friends who celebrate your strengths, cherish your uniqueness, and stand by you through thick and thin.

Don't forget that conflicts are a natural part of any relationship, and they offer valuable opportunities for growth, understanding, and connection. Trust yourself, trust your friends, and navigate the ups and downs of friendship with grace, resilience, and unwavering self-belief.

Overcoming Anxiety and Stress

Practice Mindfulness

Ground Yourself in the Present Moment: Anxiety often thrives on worries about the future or regrets about the past.

Mindfulness invites you to anchor yourself firmly in the present moment, where peace and clarity reside.

Take a few deep breaths and tune into your senses—notice the sights, sounds, smells, and sensations around you. By grounding yourself in the here and now, you can quiet the noise of anxious thoughts and cultivate a sense of calm and presence.

Practice Mindful Breathing: Your breath is a powerful anchor that can guide you back to the present moment whenever anxiety threatens to pull you away.

Take a few moments throughout your day to focus on your breath—notice the rise and fall of your chest, the sensation of air entering and leaving your nostrils. As you breathe deeply and intentionally, allow yourself to let go of tension and stress with each exhale, and invite in a sense of peace and relaxation with each inhale.

Engage in Body Scan Meditation: Your body is a sacred vessel that carries you through life's journey, and tuning into its sensations can be a powerful way to cultivate mindfulness and self-awareness.

 Practice a body scan meditation by gently directing your attention to each part of your body, starting from your toes and working your way up to the crown of your head. Notice any areas of tension, discomfort, or sensation, and breathe into those areas with compassion and acceptance.

Cultivate Gratitude: In the midst of anxiety and stress, it can be easy to lose sight of the blessings that surround you.

Cultivate a spirit of gratitude by taking time each day to reflect on the things you're thankful for—big or small.

Keep a gratitude journal where you can jot down three things you're grateful for each day, or simply take a few moments before bed to mentally list the things that brought you joy and appreciation throughout the day. By shifting your focus from what's lacking to what's abundant, you can cultivate a mindset of abundance and contentment.

Practice Mindful Movement: Movement is a beautiful expression of mindfulness, allowing you to connect with your body and breath in a fluid, harmonious dance.

Engage in activities like yoga, tai chi, or walking meditation that invite you to move with intention and awareness. Notice the sensation of your muscles stretching and contracting, the rhythm of your breath syncing with your movements, and the feeling of groundedness and vitality that arises as you move mindfully through space.

Respond, Don't React: When faced with challenging situations or triggers for anxiety, mindfulness empowers you to respond with grace and wisdom rather than react impulsively.

Take a pause before responding, allowing yourself to check in with your thoughts, emotions, and values. Ask yourself, "Is this response in alignment with my truest self? Is it serving my highest good?" By cultivating this pause, you can break free from automatic reactions and choose intentional responses that honor your well-being and integrity.

Find Moments of Stillness: In the hustle and bustle of daily life, it's essential to carve out moments of stillness and silence to nourish your spirit and replenish your energy.

Set aside time each day for mindfulness practices like meditation, journaling, or simply sitting in quiet contemplation. Create a sacred space where you can retreat from the noise of the world and reconnect with your inner sanctuary of peace and tranquility.

Manage Your Time Wisely

Set Priorities: When it feels like there aren't enough hours in the day to juggle school, extracurricular activities, social commitments, and personal hobbies, setting priorities is your secret weapon.

Take some time to reflect on your values, goals, and aspirations, and identify the tasks and activities that are most important to you. By focusing your time and energy on your top priorities, you can create a sense of purpose and direction that helps alleviate anxiety and stress.

Create a Schedule: A well-planned schedule is your roadmap to success, helping you stay organized, focused, and on track with your goals and commitments.

Invest in a planner, digital calendar, or time management app that works for you, and use it to map out your days, weeks, and months with precision and clarity.

Block out time for essential tasks like studying, attending classes, and completing assignments, as well as time for self-care, relaxation, and leisure activities.

By creating a balanced schedule that honors both your responsibilities and your well-being, you can reduce stress and create space for joy and fulfillment in your life.

Break Tasks into Manageable Chunks: Feeling overwhelmed by a mountain of homework or a daunting project?

Break it down into smaller, more manageable chunks, and tackle them one at a time. Set specific, achievable goals for each task, and focus on making progress rather than aiming for perfection. Celebrate your accomplishments along the way, no matter how small, and trust that each step forward brings you closer to your goals.

Use Time-Blocking Techniques: Time-blocking is a powerful time management technique that involves allocating specific blocks of time for different tasks or activities.

Divide your day into blocks of time dedicated to different areas of your life, such as academics, extracurriculars, self-care, and relaxation. Set boundaries around each time block and commit to focusing exclusively on the task at hand during that time.

By compartmentalizing your time in this way, you can increase productivity, reduce distractions, and maintain a healthy work-life balance.

Practice the Two-Minute Rule: When it comes to managing your time effectively, sometimes it's the small, seemingly insignificant tasks that can pile up and cause stress.

Enter the two-minute rule: if a task can be completed in two minutes or less, do it immediately. Whether it's responding to an email, tidying up your workspace, or making a quick phone call, tackling these small tasks right away can prevent them from snowballing into bigger sources of stress later on.

Learn to Say No: As a teen girl with a multitude of interests, commitments, and obligations, it's easy to fall into the trap of overcommitment and people-pleasing.

But here's the thing: your time and energy are precious resources, and it's okay to say no to things that don't align with your priorities or values.

Practice setting boundaries and politely declining requests or invitations that don't serve your best interests. Remember, saying no to others is saying yes to yourself and your well-being.

Take Regular Breaks: In the midst of a busy schedule, it's essential to prioritize self-care and relaxation to prevent burnout and overwhelm.

Schedule regular breaks throughout your day to rest, recharge, and rejuvenate your mind, body, and soul.

Whether it's taking a short walk, practicing mindfulness, or simply closing your eyes and taking a few deep breaths, find activities that help you relax and unwind and incorporate them into your daily routine.

Practice Self-Compassion

Extend Kindness to Yourself: When anxiety and stress come knocking at your door, it's easy to fall into the trap of self-criticism and self-judgment.

But here's the secret: you are worthy of love, kindness, and compassion, exactly as you are. Treat yourself with the same tenderness and understanding you would offer to a cherished friend, and remember that you are doing the best you can with the tools and resources you have.

Be gentle with yourself, my dear friend, and know that you are enough, just as you are.

Practice Self-Care: Self-compassion is about honoring your needs and prioritizing your well-being, especially during times of stress and uncertainty. Carve out time each day for self-care activities that nourish your mind, body, and soul, whether it's taking a bubble bath, going for a nature walk, or curling up with a good book.

Listen to your inner wisdom and give yourself permission to rest, recharge, and replenish your energy in whatever way feels most nurturing to you.

Release Perfectionism: As a teen girl navigating the pressures of school, social life, and personal growth, it's easy to fall into the trap of perfectionism—the belief that you must be flawless and achieve impossible standards to be worthy of love and acceptance. But here's the truth: perfection is an illusion, and embracing your imperfections is the key to true freedom and self-acceptance.

Embrace your mistakes, celebrate your progress, and allow yourself to be beautifully, wonderfully human.

Challenge Negative Self-Talk: Anxiety and stress often go hand in hand with a chorus of negative self-talk—the inner critic that whispers lies of unworthiness and inadequacy in your ear.

Challenge these negative thoughts by replacing them with compassionate, empowering affirmations that uplift and inspire you. Remind yourself of your strengths, your resilience, and your inherent worthiness, and let these truths guide you through moments of doubt and fear.

Celebrate Your Wins: In the midst of anxiety and stress, it's essential to celebrate your victories, no matter how small.

Take time to acknowledge your accomplishments, milestones, and moments of growth, and celebrate the unique journey that has brought you to this moment. Whether it's acing a test, overcoming a challenge, or simply getting out of bed in the morning, every victory is a testament to your strength, resilience, and inner beauty.

Engage in Relaxation Techniques

Practice Deep Breathing: Deep breathing is a simple yet powerful relaxation technique that can instantly calm your nervous system and ease feelings of anxiety and stress.

Find a quiet, comfortable space to sit or lie down, close your eyes, and take a few slow, deep breaths in through your nose and out through your mouth.

Allow your breath to flow naturally and effortlessly, focusing on the sensation of air entering and leaving your body.

With each breath, imagine releasing tension and worry, and inviting in a sense of peace and tranquility.

Progressive Muscle Relaxation: Progressive muscle relaxation is a wonderful technique for releasing physical tension and promoting deep relaxation throughout your body.

Start by tensing and then relaxing each muscle group in your body, one at a time, starting from your toes and working your way up to your head.

Notice the sensation of tension melting away with each release, and allow yourself to sink deeper into a state of profound relaxation and serenity.

Guided Imagery: Guided imagery is a delightful relaxation technique that uses the power of your imagination to transport you to a place of calm and tranquility.

Close your eyes and imagine yourself in a peaceful, serene setting—a lush forest, a tranquil beach, or a serene mountaintop. Engage all your senses as you visualize the sights, sounds, smells, and sensations of your chosen scene, allowing yourself to become fully immersed in the experience.

With each breath, feel yourself becoming more deeply relaxed and at ease in this magical oasis of tranquility.

Mindfulness Meditation: Mindfulness meditation is a practice of being fully present in the moment, with an attitude of openness, curiosity, and nonjudgment. Find a comfortable position to sit or lie down, close your eyes, and bring your awareness to your breath. Notice the sensation of air entering and leaving your nostrils, and allow yourself to become fully absorbed in the rhythm of your breath.

When thoughts or distractions arise, gently guide your attention back to your breath, anchoring yourself in the present moment and cultivating a sense of calm and clarity amidst the busyness of life.

Engage Your Senses: Engaging your senses is a delightful way to bring yourself into the present moment and cultivate a sense of relaxation and well-being.

Take a few moments to notice the sights, sounds, smells, tastes, and sensations around you, allowing yourself to fully experience the richness and beauty of the present moment.

Whether it's savoring a delicious piece of chocolate, listening to your favorite song, or basking in the warmth of the sun on your skin, find simple pleasures that nourish your soul and bring you joy.

Creative Expression: Engaging in creative activities like art, music, writing, or crafting can be a wonderful way to relax your mind, express your emotions, and cultivate a sense of inner peace and fulfillment.

Lose yourself in the flow of creativity as you paint, draw, write, or create, allowing yourself to tap into a deeper wellspring of inspiration and intuition.

Whether you're doodling in a sketchbook, strumming a guitar, or writing poetry, let your creativity be a source of solace and joy in times of stress and anxiety.

Nature Connection: Spending time in nature is one of the most potent relaxation techniques available to us, offering a sanctuary of peace, beauty, and tranquility amidst the hustle and bustle of modern life.

Take a leisurely stroll through a park, forest, or garden, and allow yourself to connect with the sights, sounds, smells, and sensations of the natural world.

Feel the earth beneath your feet, the sun on your face, and the gentle breeze on your skin as you immerse yourself in the healing embrace of nature.

Reach Out for Support

Lean on Trusted Friends: Your friends are more than just companions—they're your lifelines, your confidants, and your partners in crime on this wild adventure called life.

Reach out to trusted friends who you feel comfortable sharing your thoughts and feelings with, and let them know when you're struggling. Whether it's a heart-to-heart conversation over a cup of tea or a late-night chat over text, knowing that you're not alone can provide immense comfort and reassurance in times of anxiety and stress.

Turn to Family: Your family is your rock, your foundation, and your unwavering support system through thick and thin.

Don't hesitate to lean on family members who you trust and feel safe with, whether it's a parent, sibling, or relative.

Share your struggles openly and honestly with them, and allow them to offer you the love, guidance, and encouragement that only family can provide.

Remember, family is not just about blood—it's about the bonds of love and connection that unite us and carry us through life's ups and downs.

Seek Guidance from Mentors: Mentors are wise guides who have walked the path before you and can offer valuable insights, perspectives, and encouragement as you navigate the challenges of adolescence.

Whether it's a teacher, coach, counselor, or mentor figure in your community, reach out to someone you trust and admire and share your thoughts and feelings with them.

Allow them to offer you guidance, support, and a listening ear as you navigate the complexities of growing up.

Connect with Supportive Communities: There's immense strength in finding a tribe of like-minded individuals who understand and empathize with your struggles.

Seek out supportive communities both online and offline—whether it's a club, group, or online forum dedicated to a shared interest or hobby. Surround yourself with people who lift you up, inspire you, and remind you that you're not alone on this journey.

Together, you can share stories, offer support, and celebrate victories, creating a sense of belonging and connection that soothes the soul and nourishes the spirit.

Reach out to Professionals: Sometimes, anxiety and stress can feel overwhelming, and it's okay to seek professional help from a therapist, counselor, or mental health professional who specializes in supporting teens. These compassionate professionals can offer you valuable tools, insights, and strategies to help you manage anxiety and stress more effectively and reclaim control of your life.

Whether it's through individual therapy, group counseling, or online support resources, don't hesitate to reach out for help when you need it—you deserve support, understanding, and guidance on your journey to healing and wholeness.

Join Support Groups: Support groups are safe spaces where individuals can come together to share their experiences, struggles, and triumphs with others who understand and empathize.

Consider joining a support group specifically for teens dealing with anxiety and stress, where you can connect with peers who are facing similar challenges and offer each other mutual support and encouragement.

Sharing your story with others who understand can be incredibly validating and empowering, reminding you that you're not alone in your struggles and that there is hope and healing to be found in community.

Practice Vulnerability: In the midst of anxiety and stress, it can be tempting to withdraw and isolate yourself from others.

But here's the truth: vulnerability is not a weakness—it's a courageous act of self-love and self-compassion. Allow yourself to be vulnerable with those you trust, sharing your thoughts, feelings, and struggles openly and honestly.

By opening up and allowing yourself to be seen and heard, you invite others to do the same, fostering deep connections and creating a sense of belonging and support that lifts you up and carries you through life's challenges.

Overcoming anxiety and stress is a journey of self-discovery, resilience, and reclaiming your inner power, and with a little love, support, and self-care, you can emerge stronger, wiser, and more radiant than ever before.

Thriving in the Digital Age

For teen girls navigating the ever-evolving realms of social media, technology, and online communities, thriving in the digital age is about more than just mastering the latest apps and gadgets—it's about cultivating a healthy relationship with technology, harnessing its power for good, and navigating its complexities with wisdom, resilience, and integrity.

So, let's dive in and explore how you can harness the magic of the digital age to create a life of purpose, passion, and authenticity:

Embrace Digital Literacy:

In the fast-paced world of the digital age, being digitally literate is essential for navigating the online landscape with confidence and competence.

Take the time to familiarize yourself with the latest technology trends, platforms, and tools, and cultivate skills like critical thinking, media literacy, and online safety. Learn how to evaluate the credibility of information, protect your privacy and security online, and use technology responsibly and ethically. By becoming digitally literate, you can empower yourself to make informed decisions, engage with digital content mindfully, and navigate the online world with wisdom and discernment.

Cultivate a Positive Digital Identity:

Your online presence is an extension of who you are—a digital reflection of your values, interests, and personality.

Take care to cultivate a positive digital identity that aligns with your authentic self and reflects the best version of who you are. Be intentional about the content you share online, curating a feed that inspires, uplifts, and empowers others.

Use your voice and platform to spread positivity, advocate for causes you believe in, and foster meaningful connections with others.

Remember, your digital footprint has the power to shape your reputation and influence, so use it wisely and with intention.

Practice Digital Wellness:

In the age of constant connectivity and information overload, it's essential to prioritize your digital wellness and establish healthy boundaries around your technology use.

Take regular breaks from screens, engage in offline activities that nourish your mind, body, and soul, and cultivate mindfulness and presence in your digital interactions.

Set boundaries around your screen time, social media usage, and online engagement, and prioritize activities that promote balance, well-being, and connection in your life. By practicing digital wellness, you can prevent burnout, reduce stress, and create space for joy, creativity, and authentic self-expression in your online and offline experiences.

Navigate Social Media Mindfully:

Social media can be a powerful tool for connection, creativity, and self-expression, but it can also be a source of stress, comparison, and negative self-talk if used mindlessly.

Approach social media with intention and mindfulness, being mindful of how it impacts your mood, self-esteem, and overall well-being. Curate your social media feeds to include content that inspires, uplifts, and empowers you, and unfollow accounts that trigger feelings of comparison, inadequacy, or negativity.

Use social media as a platform to connect with like-minded individuals, share your passions and interests, and cultivate meaningful relationships based on authenticity, kindness, and mutual respect.

Protect Your Mental Health:

In the digital age, it's easy to get caught up in the constant stream of notifications, likes, and comments, and lose sight of your mental health and well-being. Prioritize your mental health by taking regular breaks from screens, practicing self-care activities that nourish your mind, body, and soul, and seeking support from trusted friends, family members, or mental health professionals if you're struggling.

Know that it's okay to unplug, disconnect, and prioritize your well-being over your online presence.

Your mental health is precious, and it deserves to be prioritized and protected in the digital age and beyond.

In the digital age, technology has the power to be a force for good, fostering connection, collaboration, and positive change in the world.

Use your digital platform and voice to advocate for causes you believe in, raise awareness about issues that matter to you, and amplify the voices of marginalized communities.

Engage in acts of digital activism, volunteerism, and philanthropy that make a positive impact on the world around you. By harnessing the power of technology for good, you can be a force for positive change in your community and beyond, leaving a lasting legacy of kindness, compassion, and empowerment in the digital age and beyond.

Note that technology is a tool—a canvas upon which you can paint the masterpiece of your life, expressing your unique voice, vision, and values for the world to see.

By navigating the digital age with wisdom, resilience, and integrity, you can create a life of purpose, passion, and authenticity that inspires others

and leaves a lasting impact on the
world around you.

Social Media Smarts: Balancing Online and Offline Life

For teen girls navigating the bustling landscape of social media, finding balance between their online and offline lives is key to fostering healthy habits, nurturing meaningful relationships, and thriving in both the digital and physical realms.

Now, let's explore some savvy strategies for striking the perfect balance between your digital adventures and real-life experiences:

Set Boundaries:

In the fast-paced world of social media, it's easy to get swept up in the endless scroll of notifications, likes, and comments.

But remember, you're the one in control of your online experience.

Set boundaries around your social media usage, such as limiting your screen time, designating specific times of day for checking your accounts, and taking regular breaks to disconnect and recharge.

By setting clear boundaries, you can prevent burnout, reduce stress, and create space for more meaningful interactions both online and offline.

Prioritize Quality Over Quantity:

In the age of social media, it's tempting to measure your worth by the number of followers, likes, and comments you receive.

But here's the truth: your value extends far beyond your online presence. Instead of chasing validation and approval from others, focus on cultivating quality connections and meaningful relationships with those who truly matter to you. Prioritize authenticity, kindness, and genuine engagement in your online interactions, and remember that true connection is measured not by numbers, but by the depth of the relationships you cultivate.

Practice Mindful Posting:

Before you hit that "post" button, take a moment to pause and reflect on your intentions behind sharing a particular piece of content. Ask yourself: Does this post align with my values and beliefs? Is it contributing positively to the online conversation? Am I sharing authentically and thoughtfully? By practicing mindful posting, you can ensure that your online presence reflects your true self and contributes positively to the digital community.

Curate Your Feed:

Your social media feed is like a digital mirror, reflecting back to you the content and messages you consume on a daily basis.

Take control of your digital experience by curating your feed to include content that inspires, uplifts, and empowers you. Seek out creators who share your interests, values, and passions.

Surround yourself with content that brings you joy, sparks your creativity, and fosters a sense of connection and belonging in the online world.

Balance Online and Offline Activities:

While social media offers endless opportunities for connection and entertainment, it's important to balance your online activities with offline experiences that nourish your mind, body, and soul. Make time for hobbies, interests, and activities that bring you joy and fulfillment outside of the digital realm, whether it's spending time with friends and family, exploring nature, pursuing creative projects, or engaging in physical activity.

By striking a balance between your online and offline lives, you can cultivate a sense of wholeness and well-being that enriches every aspect of your life.

Stay Safe and Secure:

In the digital age, it's essential to prioritize your online safety and security. Protect your personal information and privacy by using strong, unique passwords for your accounts, being cautious about sharing sensitive information online, and being mindful of who you connect with and interact with online.

Familiarize yourself with the privacy settings and security features of the platforms you use, and trust your instincts if something feels off or suspicious. By staying vigilant and proactive about your online safety, you can enjoy the benefits of social media while minimizing potential risks and vulnerabilities.

Be Kind and Respectful:

In the digital world, kindness is contagious, and a little bit of positivity can go a long way.

Treat others with kindness, empathy, and respect in your online interactions, and strive to create a culture of inclusivity, support, and positivity in your digital communities.

Think before you comment, and remember that behind every screen is a real person with thoughts, feelings, and experiences of their own. By spreading kindness and positivity online, you can contribute to a more compassionate and uplifting digital landscape for everyone to enjoy.

Cyberbullying Awareness and Prevention

As teen girls navigating the complexities of online interactions, it's essential to equip ourselves with the knowledge, skills, and resilience needed to stand up to cyberbullying, protect ourselves and others, and foster a culture of kindness and respect in the digital world.

Know the Signs:

Cyberbullying can take many forms, from hurtful comments and rumors to threats, harassment, and exclusion. Educate yourself about the signs of cyberbullying, such as sudden changes in mood or behavior, reluctance to go online, or withdrawal from social activities.

Be vigilant for signs that you or someone you know may be experiencing cyberbullying, and take them seriously.

Speak Up:

If you witness cyberbullying happening to someone else, don't stay silent.

Speak up and offer support to the victim, whether it's through a kind message, a show of solidarity, or reporting the abusive behavior to the appropriate authorities or platform moderators.

Remember, bystander intervention can make a world of difference in stopping cyberbullying in its tracks and showing the victim that they're not alone.

Protect Your Privacy:

In the digital age, protecting your privacy and personal information is more important than ever.

Be mindful of what you share online, and avoid posting sensitive or personal information that could be used against you by cyberbullies.

Familiarize yourself with the privacy settings and security features of the platforms you use, and take proactive steps to safeguard your online accounts and devices from potential threats.

Practice Digital Citizenship:

As digital citizens, we all have a responsibility to contribute positively to the online community and uphold ethical standards of behavior.

Treat others with kindness, empathy, and respect in your online interactions, and think twice before posting or sharing anything that could be hurtful or harmful to others.

Remember that behind every screen is a real person with thoughts, feelings, and experiences of their own.

Seek Support:

If you're experiencing cyberbullying, don't suffer in silence. Reach out to trusted friends, family members, or adults for support, and let them know what you're going through.

Consider talking to a school counselor, therapist, or mental health professional who can offer guidance, support, and strategies for coping with cyberbullying and protecting your mental and emotional well-being.

Report and Block:

Most social media platforms and online communities have policies in place to address cyberbullying and protect users from harassment and abuse.

If you're being cyberbullied, don't hesitate to report the abusive behavior to the platform administrators or moderators, and consider blocking the person responsible to prevent further contact. Remember that reporting cyberbullying is not about getting someone in trouble—it's about protecting yourself and others from harm and creating a safer, more inclusive online environment for everyone.

Educate and Advocate:

Raise awareness about cyberbullying and its harmful effects by educating others about the issue and advocating for change in your school, community, and online platforms.

Organize awareness campaigns, workshops, or events to promote cyberbullying prevention and empower your peers to stand up against bullying in all its forms. By shining a light on cyberbullying and promoting a culture of kindness and respect, you can help create a world where all teens can thrive free from fear and harassment.

Be aware that you have the power to make a difference in the fight against cyberbullying, both in your own life and in the lives of others.

Together, we can create a world where kindness triumphs over cruelty, empathy conquers hate, and every teen girl can thrive free from the shadow of cyberbullying.

Excelling in School and Beyond

Study Tips for Success

As a teenager, navigating the whirlwind of schoolwork, extracurricular activities, and personal pursuits, mastering the art of effective studying is key to achieving your goals, realizing your dreams, and carving out a bright future filled with endless possibilities.

Create a Study Schedule:

One of the most powerful tools in your academic arsenal is a well-crafted study schedule. Take the time to map out your week, allocating dedicated blocks of time for studying, homework, and revision.

Be realistic about your commitments and prioritize tasks based on their importance and deadlines. By creating a study schedule and sticking to it, you can maximize your productivity, manage your time effectively, and stay on top of your academic responsibilities.

Find Your Learning Style:

We all have unique ways of processing information and learning new concepts. Take the time to identify your preferred learning style—whether it's visual, auditory, kinesthetic, or a combination of different modalities—and tailor your study techniques accordingly.

Experiment with different study methods, such as visual aids, flashcards, mnemonics, or hands-on activities, and discover what works best for you.

By aligning your study strategies with your learning style, you can enhance your understanding, retention, and recall of course material.

Stay Organized:

A cluttered workspace can lead to a cluttered mind, making it difficult to focus and concentrate on your studies.

Keep your study area tidy and organized, with all the materials and resources you need readily accessible.

Invest in a planner, calendar, or digital organization tool to keep track of assignments, deadlines, and important dates, and use color-coding or labeling systems to streamline your notes and materials. By maintaining an organized study environment, you can minimize distractions, boost productivity, and create space for focused learning.

Break It Down:

Tackling large tasks or assignments can feel overwhelming, leading to procrastination and avoidance.

Break down your study sessions into smaller, more manageable chunks, and focus on one task or concept at a time.

Set specific, achievable goals for each study session, and reward yourself with breaks or rewards as you make progress. By breaking down your study sessions into bite-sized pieces, you can make studying feel more manageable and less daunting, leading to greater efficiency and success.

Practice Active Learning:

Passive studying, such as re-reading notes or textbooks, can be ineffective for long-term retention and understanding.

Instead, engage in active learning techniques that require you to actively process and apply the information you're studying. Practice active recall by quizzing yourself on key concepts, use spaced repetition to reinforce your learning over time, and teach the material to a friend or family member to solidify your understanding.

By actively engaging with the material, you can deepen your comprehension, strengthen your memory, and achieve mastery in your studies.

Take Care of Yourself:

Your well-being is the foundation of your academic success. Prioritize self-care activities that nourish your mind, body, and soul, such as getting enough sleep, eating nutritious meals, staying hydrated, and engaging in regular exercise.

Take breaks when you need them, and listen to your body's signals when it's time to rest and recharge. Remember that a healthy, balanced lifestyle is essential for maintaining focus, concentration, and motivation in your studies.

Seek Support:

Don't hesitate to reach out for help when you need it. Whether it's asking a teacher for clarification on a difficult concept, joining a study group to collaborate with peers, or seeking tutoring or academic support services, there are plenty of resources available to help you succeed.

Don't let pride or fear hold you back from seeking support—remember that asking for help is a sign of strength, not weakness, and that there's always someone willing to lend a helping hand on your academic journey.

Note that academic success is not about perfection—it's about progress, growth, and the journey of self-discovery and learning. By implementing these strategies into your study routine, you can unlock your full potential, conquer any academic challenge that comes your way, and embark on a journey of lifelong learning and achievement.

Navigating Love and Relationships

When going through the complexities of romance, friendship, and self-discovery as a teenage girl, it's normal to feel excited, curious, and maybe even a little bit nervous about what lies ahead. But fear not, because you're not alone on this journey.

Together, we'll explore some savvy strategies for navigating love and relationships with confidence, authenticity, and grace:

Know Yourself:

Before you can embark on a journey of love and relationships with others, it's essential to know and love yourself first.

Take the time to explore your interests, passions, and values, and embrace the unique qualities that make you who you are.

Get to know your likes and dislikes, your strengths and weaknesses, and what makes your heart sing with joy. By cultivating a strong sense of self-awareness and self-love, you'll be better equipped to navigate the ups and downs of love and relationships with grace and authenticity.

Set Healthy Boundaries:

 Boundaries are like personal guardrails that help protect your emotional well-being and preserve your sense of self in relationships.

Take the time to establish clear boundaries for yourself in romantic relationships, friendships, and interactions with others, and communicate them openly and assertively with those around you.

Respect your own boundaries and those of others, and be willing to advocate for your needs and desires in a respectful and compassionate manner. Know that setting healthy boundaries is an act of self-care and self-respect, and it's essential for maintaining healthy, fulfilling relationships.

Communicate Openly:

Effective communication is the cornerstone of any healthy relationship. Practice open, honest, and respectful communication with your romantic partner, friends, and family members, and be willing to express your thoughts, feelings, and needs openly and authentically.

Listen actively to what others have to say, and strive to understand their perspectives and emotions without judgment or criticism.

By fostering open communication in your relationships, you can build trust, deepen connection, and navigate conflicts and challenges with greater ease and understanding.

Trust Your Instincts:

Your instincts are powerful guides that can help you navigate the complexities of love and relationships with wisdom and intuition.

Trust your gut feelings and intuition when it comes to making decisions about who to trust, who to date, and how to navigate challenging situations in your relationships.

Pay attention to red flags or warning signs that indicate when something doesn't feel right, and be willing to listen to your inner voice, even if it goes against external pressure or expectations. Remember that you are the ultimate authority on your own life and relationships, and your instincts are there to guide you towards what's best for you.

Prioritize Mutual Respect:

Respect is the foundation of any healthy relationship, whether it's romantic, platonic, or familial.

Treat others with kindness, empathy, and compassion, and expect the same in return. Respect each other's boundaries, opinions, and autonomy, and strive to create a relationship dynamic built on equality, trust, and mutual understanding. If you ever find yourself in a situation where your boundaries are being violated or your dignity is being disrespected, don't hesitate to speak up and advocate for yourself.

Know that you deserve to be treated with respect and dignity in all your relationships, and don't settle for anything less.

Take Things Slow:

In the early stages of dating, it's important to take things slow and allow the relationship to unfold naturally over time. Resist the urge to rush into things or force the relationship to progress faster than it's ready for. Take the time to get to know each other on a deeper level, build trust and emotional intimacy, and explore your compatibility as partners. Trust your instincts and listen to your heart, and let the relationship evolve at its own pace.

Stay True to Yourself:

In the midst of dating, it's easy to lose sight of who you are and what you want in a relationship. Stay true to yourself and your values, and don't compromise your authenticity for the sake of pleasing your partner or fitting into their expectations. Embrace your unique qualities, quirks, and interests, and celebrate what makes you who you are.

It is important to bear in mind that the right person will love and appreciate you for exactly who you are, flaws and all.

Embrace Growth and Change:

Love and relationships are dynamic and ever-evolving, just like you. Embrace the journey of growth and change that comes with being in relationships, and be open to learning, evolving, and growing together with your partner or friends.

Celebrate each other's successes, support each other through challenges, and cherish the moments of growth and transformation that come with navigating love and relationships as a teenage girl.

Note that every relationship has its ups and downs, and it's the journey of growth and learning together that ultimately strengthens the bonds of love and friendship.

Bear in mind that love and relationships are a journey, not a destination, and every experience—whether it's a moment of joy, a lesson learned, or a challenge overcome—is an opportunity for growth and self-discovery.

Trust yourself, follow your heart, and embrace the adventure of love and relationships with grace and confidence.

Financial Fitness for the Future

Money Management Basics

Understand the Basics: The first step in mastering money is to understand the basics of personal finance.

Take the time to familiarize yourself with fundamental concepts like budgeting, saving, spending, and investing, and learn how to make smart financial decisions that align with your goals and values. Don't forget that knowledge is power, and by educating yourself about money management, you can take control of your financial future and build a solid foundation for success.

Create a Budget:

A budget is your roadmap to financial success, helping you track your income, expenses, and savings goals with precision and clarity.

Take the time to create a budget that reflects your income, expenses, and financial goals, and allocate your money wisely to cover essentials like food, housing, transportation, and entertainment, while also setting aside funds for savings and emergencies. Be realistic about your spending habits and financial goals, and adjust your budget as needed to stay on track and achieve your objectives.

Save, Save, Save:

 Saving money is one of the most powerful tools for building wealth and achieving financial security over time.

Make saving a priority by setting aside a portion of your income each month for short-term goals like buying a new gadget or going on vacation, as well as long-term goals like building an emergency fund or saving for college. Consider opening a savings account or investment account to help your money grow over time, and explore opportunities for maximizing your savings through strategies like compound interest and dollar-cost averaging.

Live Within Your Means:

It can be tempting to spend beyond your means, especially when faced with peer pressure or societal expectations to keep up with the latest trends and fads. But living within your means is essential for maintaining financial stability and avoiding debt and financial hardship down the road. Practice mindful spending by distinguishing between needs and wants, prioritizing purchases that align with your values and goals, and avoiding impulse buys or unnecessary expenses that can derail your budget.

Be Smart About Credit:

Credit can be a valuable tool for building financial independence and achieving your goals, but it can also be a double-edged sword if mismanaged. Take the time to learn about credit cards, loans, and other forms of credit, and understand how they work, including interest rates, fees, and repayment terms.

Use credit responsibly by paying your bills on time, keeping your credit utilization low, and avoiding excessive debt or frivolous spending. Note that good credit habits today can pave the way for a bright financial future tomorrow.

Invest in Yourself:

As a teenager, investing in yourself is one of the best investments you can make for your future success and happiness. Take advantage of opportunities for personal and professional growth, whether it's through education, training, hobbies, or extracurricular activities.

Invest in developing your skills, talents, and passions, and explore opportunities for building a rewarding and fulfilling career that aligns with your interests and values.

Investing in yourself is an investment that pays dividends for a lifetime.

Invest Wisely:

Investing is one of the most powerful tools for building wealth and achieving financial independence over the long term.

Take the time to educate yourself about different investment options, such as stocks, bonds, mutual funds, real estate, and retirement accounts, and explore opportunities for diversifying your investment portfolio to minimize risk and maximize returns.

Consider working with a financial advisor or investment professional to develop a personalized investment strategy that aligns with your goals, risk tolerance, and time horizon. Remember that investing is a marathon, not a sprint, and patience and discipline are key to long-term success.

Build Multiple Streams of Income:

Building financial independence requires more than just a single source of income—it requires diversifying your income streams and creating multiple sources of revenue that can support your financial goals and lifestyle.

Explore opportunities for generating passive income through investments, rental properties, royalties, or online businesses, and consider ways to leverage your skills, talents, and interests to create additional income streams.

By building multiple streams of income, you can create a stable and resilient financial foundation that can weather any storm and support your dreams and aspirations.

Practice Patience and Persistence:

Building financial independence is a journey, not a destination, and it requires patience, persistence, and perseverance to achieve your goals. Stay focused on your long-term vision and keep moving forward, even in the face of setbacks or challenges.

Celebrate your progress along the way, no matter how small, and remember that every step you take towards financial independence brings you closer to living the life of your dreams.

Trust yourself, believe in your abilities, and never give up on your quest for financial empowerment and freedom.

Seek Guidance and Support:

Don't be afraid to seek guidance and support from trusted adults, mentors, or financial professionals as you navigate the complexities of money management.

Reach out to parents, teachers, or other knowledgeable individuals for advice, resources, and guidance on topics like budgeting, saving, investing, and financial planning.

Consider enrolling in a financial literacy course or workshop to expand your knowledge and skills, and explore opportunities for mentorship and networking with experts in the field. Always know that you're not alone on your financial journey, and there are plenty of resources available to help you succeed.

Preparing for College and Beyond

Define Your Goals:

Before diving into the college preparation process, take some time to reflect on your goals, passions, and aspirations.

What are you passionate about? What subjects or activities bring you joy and fulfillment? What do you envision for your future career and personal growth? By clarifying your goals and priorities, you can create a roadmap for success that aligns with your values and aspirations.

Explore Your Options:

Once you have a clear understanding of your goals, it's time to explore your options for higher education and beyond.

Research different colleges, universities, and vocational programs that offer programs and resources aligned with your interests and career goals.

Consider factors such as location, size, academic offerings, extracurricular activities, and campus culture to find the best fit for your needs and preferences.

Build Your Skills:

College and beyond require a diverse set of skills, including critical thinking, communication, problem-solving, and time management.

Take advantage of opportunities to develop these skills both inside and outside the classroom.

Participate in extracurricular activities, volunteer work, internships, or part-time jobs that allow you to gain hands-on experience and build valuable skills that will serve you well in college and beyond.

Academic Excellence:

Maintaining strong academic performance is essential for college admission and future success.

Take your studies seriously and strive for excellence in your coursework, exams, and standardized tests.

Seek out challenging courses that stretch your abilities and demonstrate your academic rigor to college admissions officers. Don't hesitate to ask for help or seek additional support if you're struggling in a particular subject—remember, it's okay to ask for help when you need it.

Plan Financially:

College can be a significant financial investment, so it's essential to plan ahead and explore your options for funding your education.

Research scholarships, grants, and financial aid opportunities available to you, and explore different ways to save money for college, such as opening a savings account or starting a college fund. Consider the cost of tuition, fees, room and board, textbooks, and other expenses when planning your college budget, and be proactive about exploring options for reducing costs and maximizing financial aid.

Cultivate Relationships:

Building strong relationships with teachers, mentors, peers, and professionals can provide valuable support and guidance as you navigate the college preparation process and beyond.

Seek out mentors who can offer advice and insight based on their own experiences, and cultivate relationships with teachers and counselors who can provide academic support and guidance.

Connect with peers who share your interests and aspirations, and explore opportunities for networking and collaboration within your community.

Embrace Personal Growth:

College and beyond are not just about academic achievement—they're also about personal growth and self-discovery. Embrace opportunities for personal growth and self-reflection, and take the time to explore your interests, passions, and values.

Engage in activities that challenge you, push you out of your comfort zone, and help you develop as a well-rounded individual.

Be aware that college is not just about preparing for a career—it's about preparing for life.

Stay Resilient:

The college preparation process can be challenging and overwhelming at times, but remember that setbacks and obstacles are a natural part of any journey.

Stay resilient in the face of adversity, and don't let setbacks deter you from pursuing your goals and dreams.

Learn from your mistakes, adapt to challenges, and keep moving forward with determination, perseverance, and unwavering self-belief.

Stay True to Yourself:

Above all, stay true to yourself and your values as you navigate the college preparation process and beyond. Don't let external pressures or expectations dictate your path— follow your heart and pursue your passions with courage, conviction, and authenticity.

Trust yourself, believe in your abilities, and know that you have the power to create a future that's uniquely yours.

Note that the road to college and beyond is filled with twists and turns, but with determination, perseverance, and a little bit of savvy, you can navigate the journey with grace and confidence. Trust yourself, follow your dreams, and prepare to embark

on the adventure of a lifetime. The

world is waiting for you—go forth and

conquer it!

Conclusion

Congratulations, dear reader, on reaching the conclusion of this empowering journey!

As you close the final pages of this book, I hope you're feeling inspired, empowered, and ready to embark on your own path to greatness.

Throughout these chapters, we've explored a myriad of topics, from navigating friendships and relationships to mastering money management and building a bright future filled with possibility. But more than just practical advice and savvy strategies, this book has been a beacon of empowerment—a guiding light illuminating the path to your true potential.

As a teenage girl navigating the complexities of adolescence and beyond, you possess a unique blend of strength, resilience, and boundless potential.

You are capable of achieving anything you set your mind to, overcoming any obstacle in your path, and creating a life that's rich with meaning, purpose, and fulfillment. But remember, true empowerment isn't just about achieving external success—it's about embracing who you are, honoring your worth, and living authentically in alignment with your values and dreams.

As you journey forward from these pages, I encourage you to hold fast to the lessons learned, the wisdom gained, and the dreams ignited within your heart.

Embrace the power of self-love, self-belief, and self-discovery as your guiding principles, and trust in your ability to create the life you envision for yourself. Surround yourself with supportive friends, mentors, and role models who lift you up, cheer you on, and remind you of your inherent worth and potential.

www.ingramcontent.com/pod-product-compliance
Lightning Source LLC
Chambersburg PA
CBHW051600250726
48653CB00004BA/1248